The Natural Hair Handbook: Everything You Need to Know About Natural Hair

by Shawntay Jones

Disclaimer:

Dedication:

This book is dedicated to all my natural-hair wearing sisters out there. Keep it natural and keep it looking good!

Contents

Introduction

With all of the information out there on natural hair care, things can get a bit overwhelming. Everywhere you turn, there's a book, blog or website telling you what you should and shouldn't do with natural hair. It can be a bit confusing, to say the least.

This book was written with the beginner in mind. I'm going to assume you know next to nothing about natural hair and start from there. That's not to say there's nothing of value in this book for seasoned vets. Quite the contrary, in fact. This book will be a good refresher and you might actually learn a thing or two.

The journey into the world of natural hair can be a confusing and tumultuous ride, especially in the beginning stages. The intent of this book is to take as much of the guesswork out of it as possible. I want you to finish this book with the knowledge you need to make smart, informed decisions about your hair.

Going natural is a journey with no single endpoint you end up at. Everyone walks their own path and has their own experiences they have to deal with. What works for you may not be acceptable to the next person in line. You may see people who take caring for their hair to an extreme you may not be willing to go to. On the other hand, you may be one of the people who are willing to spend countless hours caring for your hair.

At its core, natural hair is about acceptance. You accept the fact that your natural hair is bold and beautiful. In turn, you expect the world to accept your newfound natural state. I find it humorous (and a little sad) when I check in on my favorite natural hair forums to find naturals arguing and bickering over petty stuff. It's all about acceptance, folks. We need to be willing to accept that not everyone is going to be willing to go on the same journey we're on. Our paths will all be different.

In the end, aren't we all shooting for the same thing? We're embracing our natural beauty. By going natural, we're telling the world we're proud of who we are and that they'd better be willing to accept us in our natural state. Go big, go bold, go beautiful . . . Go natural.

What Does It Mean to "Go Natural"?

Going natural is the act of transitioning your hair from a relaxed hairstyle back to its natural state. Natural hair is hair that is not relaxed, straightened or otherwise altered by chemical or mechanical means.

There is no single right way to make the transition from relaxed to natural. What's important is that you've made the decision to do it.

You might decide to simply let your hair grow out and slowly but surely eliminate the relaxed hair by cutting it a bit at a time at regular intervals. If you decide to go this route, you're going to have to figure out a way to manage your *line of demarcation*. This is the point where your old relaxed hair and your new natural hair meet.

Your hair will be healthier and shinier on the natural side than it will be on the relaxed side. Your hair takes a beating when it's straightened. Just how much damage you've done doesn't become evident until you start letting it grow out and are able to compare the new healthy hair to the old damaged hair. Once hair is damaged, it can't be repaired. There's no magic shampoo or treatment that's going to make your old hair match your new hair in color and texture.

That's why some people decide to go with what's called *The Big Chop*. If you've been considering going natural for a while, you're probably aware of what The Big Chop is. It's the fastest way to go natural. It's also the easiest, at least from a manageability standpoint. When you do The Big Chop, you cut off all of your hair and start fresh. That's right; you cut your hair off—all of it. We'll cover The Big Chop in a later chapter. For now, all you need to know is what it is.

Making the Decision to Go Natural

You may have been thinking about going natural for quite some time. It's a big decision, and one many women ponder for a long time before finally pulling the trigger.

What will people think? Will I catch any blowback? Will it affect my life at home? Will it affect my career?

There are a number of reasons you may be having second thoughts. This is something you've got to sort through on your own; just know that you're not alone. The questions you're asking yourself are the same ones tens of thousands of people before you have struggled with.

Let's take a look at some of the more common questions. If yours aren't on here, get online and search out an active natural hair forum. Sign up and ask your question. I'm sure you'll find plenty of other people who had the same questions you do before they went natural.

Will Going Natural Negatively Impact My Professional Life?

I'm not going to lie to you or sugarcoat things here. There are a select few people who think natural hair looks unprofessional. If your boss happens to be one of those people, it could negatively impact your ability to advance your career. There are some people who are closed-minded an judge a person based on some negative misconception they have about natural hair.

That said; in this day and age those people tend to be few and far between. There are plenty of companies out there with plenty of bosses who won't care what you do with your hair as long as you show up to work looking neat and professional. You may be pleasantly surprised at the way your coworkers react to your new hair. I've personally heard numerous stories from people who were terrified to go to work and show their new natural who got to work and started getting *compliments* from their coworkers.

The key here is to stay neat and professional. If you show up to work with your hair half-braided and unkempt, you're going to get a lot of sideways glances. Those looks aren't from people wondering why you have natural hair; they're from people wondering why you didn't care enough to finish doing your hair. There's a big difference.

Going natural doesn't mean going rogue and never having to touch your hair again. It means embracing your new hair and finding new styles that work for you and fit in with your personal and professional life. You have to be able to step back and look at your place of work and then choose a hair style that fits your profession. If you work at a law office and you show up with braids that are died bright pink, you're probably not going to fit in. On the other hand, if you work as a bartender at a trendy new club, the hot pink braids may fit right in.

Natural hair can be done in a number of ways that look neat, well-kept and professional. Choose one of those styles and going natural shouldn't be a problem at all. If it is, it's time to start asking yourself whether you're working at the right company. Do you really want to try to further your career at a company that discriminates against you because you want to have your hair in the style that it naturally grows in?

Your hair color, style and texture have nothing to do with your talent and ability. It stands to reason that a company willing to discriminate against someone with natural hair already has other preconceived notions about black people in general. I, for one, refuse to work for a company that won't accept me in my natural state.

If more people wore their hair naturally, there would be less backlash against those who do. People tend to be afraid of and shun things they aren't familiar with. If more people had natural hair, it would become a non-issue because it wouldn't stick out like a sore thumb.

What Will People Say?

When it comes to your new natural hair, everyone is going to have an opinion at first. They're either going to love it or hate it. You're going to have to roll with the punches. It'll pass once people start getting used to your new hairstyle.

Oddly enough, you may find that the people who show the most disdain toward your new hairstyle are the ones you'd think would embrace it most. That's right; other black people might be your biggest critic. There's widespread disdain in the elderly black community against those of us who have decided to explore our natural roots.

If you've ever been privy to a conversation about natural hair when it's about someone else, you know what to expect. Natural women tend to get grouped together and thrown into one of a handful of "all women with natural hair are this way" stereotypes. The people who stereotype you will assume you're either low-maintenance, trying to get back at the man or lazy and have given up on trying to get ahead in life.

I've found it's the elderly people in my community who speak out the most vehemently about natural hair. They have no problem stating their opinion loudly and to anyone who'll listen. I just grin and bear it. It helps to remember that they grew up in different times and it was to their benefit at times to try to blend in and conform.

In order to give you an idea of what to expect, I've collected a handful of questions and statements people have actually been asked or told. Some are funny, some are mildly amusing and some are just sad:

- "Is that your real hair or a wig?"
- "You mean all that hair is yours?"
- "I didn't know you were black and angry."
- "You have natural hair. You must be low-maintenance."
- "I'm jealous of your hair. You must have Indian in your family."
- "Look at all that hair. It would be beautiful if you got it permed."
- "You look just like Whoopi Goldberg."
- "You look so exotic. Are you from Africa?"
- "I could never go natural. My hair's too black."
- "You cut all of your hair off? It used to be so beautiful."
- "Is that a weave? It looks so real."
- "Have you been in America long?"
- "You need to do something about that hair, girl."
- "Your hair's gone. Do…Do you have cancer?"
- "You decided to throw in the towel, eh?"

For the most part, the comments will be well-intentioned, if not a little opinionated. Some of the worst comments I've heard were actually meant to be compliments. Take the Whoopi Goldberg comment for example. A friend of mine heard that one from an elderly white woman who she'd just met. The woman was truly shocked when my friend didn't eat that comment up.

Don't get me wrong; it isn't going to be all bad. You'll get plenty of compliments on your new hair style, too. There are going to be just as many people who are going to love your hair as there will be detractors.

Everyone is going to have an opinion on you going natural and there isn't much you're going to be able to do to change their opinion. And you know what? It really doesn't matter what anyone thinks or says as long as you're happy with your choice. Going natural is something you do for yourself, not for anyone else.

What Will People Think?

The answer to this question is anything and everything. You dream it up; there's probably someone out there that will think it about your natural hair. People are very opinionated when it comes to natural hairstyles. It's a love or hate thing, with only a select few in the middle with no opinion one way or the other.

My answer to this question is *why do you care so much what other people will think?*

It's your hair. It's on your head. You can do what you want with it and, as long as you're not doing something wild and destructive, you're going to be fine.

No matter what haircut you get, no matter how you style your hair, no matter how hard you try to please everyone, you are going to have people that like your hair and people that don't like your hair. In the end, what really matters is that you like your hair. If you're happier with natural hair than you are with relaxed hair, then by all means go natural.

People are going to think what they will. If they're shallow enough to think differently of you because your hair has a different texture to it, then they aren't the type of people you should worry about anyhow. Do what's right for you and let the cards fall where they will.

Do Men Like Natural Hair?

No matter what you do to your body and your hair, there are going to be men who like it and men who don't.

Case in point, I have a girlfriend who was pushing 200 pounds who went on a diet because she was tired of being overweight and thought losing weight would help her attract better men. She lost 75 pounds and was looking fit and trim and feeling pretty good about herself. She finally got up the nerve to ask a man out who she'd had her eye on for a while and was promptly turned down. When she asked why, the man told her he preferred a woman with some meat on her bones.

When it comes, some men like and prefer natural hair, some men don't like it and some don't care one way or the other.

A survey of black men in the United States would more than likely reveal more men have a preference for straight hair over natural hair. While many men claim to be enlightened enough not to care, they go for the girl with the straight hair over the girl with the natural hair time and time again. There are a number of reasons for this, not the least of which is mainstream media's tendency to portray women with relaxed hair as the epitome of beauty. How often do you see natural-haired goddesses portrayed as beautiful on TV?

The good news is there are a group of men of all races who are enlightened enough to approve of and like natural hair. You might have to look a little harder to find a man who loves your hair, but they're out there. They're also less likely to be hung up on your looks and more likely to accept you for who you are on the inside—not that natural hair isn't beautiful. It is, and you are—and you'll be beautiful no matter what hair style you have.

Will you be able to land a good man with natural hair? Absolutely. There are millions of naturals the world over who have. Will it be easy? That depends on your definition of easy. Good men are hard to find no matter what hairstyle you have.

Will My Significant Other Like It?

Maybe, maybe not. The only way to find out for sure is to ask—or just cut it and deal with the fallout. I'd suggest at least mentioning it a couple times and trying to feel your partner out first. That way, at least you can make an informed decision.

If he doesn't like the idea of you going natural, you have a tough decision to make. You can forget about going natural, which isn't a good option for you but may prevent some strife in your relationship, or you can go natural and try to condition your man to the point where he likes it—or at least accepts it.

At the very least, you should try to talk it over with him to find out what it is he doesn't like. You might be surprised to find it's something the two of you can work out amicably. A common complaint amongst men who don't like natural hair is that they think it's going to have a rough texture. If you use the right hair care products for your hair, your hair will be soft and supple.

The biggest reason your man won't like the idea of you going natural is because men are creatures of comfort and are more comfortable with something they know than something that's foreign to them. You've had relaxed hair since your man met you and he's grown accustomed to you having relaxed hair. He isn't going to understand your newfound desire to go natural.

Most men aren't as concerned with their wives or girlfriends going natural as they are about them looking good. As long as you do your hair nice and look cute, your man probably won't care. I've heard stories from girlfriends who have long-time boyfriends who didn't even notice when they went natural. While I would never advocate lying to your significant other about your hair, it may be worth trying going natural by letting your hair grow out without saying anything to see if he notices. Continue doing your hair nice and slowly transition into cute natural hairstyles.

Those of you planning on doing The Big Chop aren't going to be able to be as subtle. You need to talk to your man. You'd better believe he's going to notice when you come home with hair shorter than his. He's probably not going to like it—and he's going to be upset you didn't mention it to him before you did it.

Remember, this is a journey. It isn't just a journey for you—it's also a journey for your man.

He's going to have to learn to live with the new you and it may take some time for him to adjust to your new natural hair. Give him some time and he might just surprise you. As long as you're happy and comfortable with your hair, he should be, too. If not, he may not be the right person for you to spend the rest of your life with. It's important that we keep our husbands and boyfriends happy, but at what cost. I draw the line at sacrificing my well-being over something as trivial as a decision about hair.

Your Hair

Before we get started on going natural and maintaining natural hair, it's important that you understand a few facts about hair in general. This section of the book is going to break down the science behind your hair and how it grows.

You don't need to remember all of it, but a basic knowledge of hair and when and how it grows will help you understand what's going on with your hair. A lot of "problems" people have with their hair are simply misunderstandings in regard to the stages of growth their hair is in. Understanding the stages of growth allows you to properly assess any issues that may arise.

Hair is made largely of a protein called *keratin*, which is the same material your fingernails and toenails are made up of. It's dead material, so that's why you don't feel anything when you cut it—or when you treat it with harsh chemicals. The body gives no indication that you're damaging your hair. You don't feel it, and since it happens slowly over a long period of time, you don't notice the damage until it's pretty bad. You'll notice it when you start growing your new hair out, and you're probably going to be surprised at just how bad the damage is.

Your hair is made up of approximately 91% keratin and 9% moisture. The moisture is in the form of natural oils called *lipids* and water.

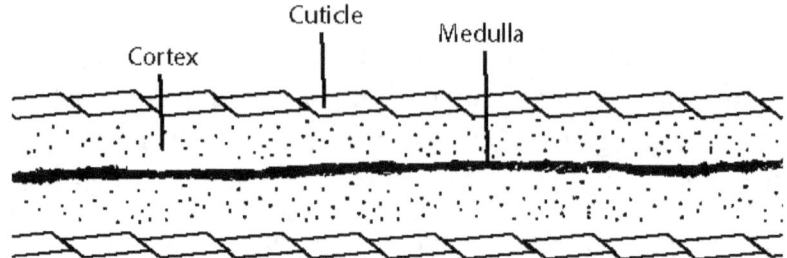

Hair has three layers:

- **Medula.** The medula is the innermost layer. It's made of soft, spongy cells and is typically 1/3 the width of the strand of hair. The medula can run the entire length of the hair or it might just be found in small fragments along the length of the hair.
- **Cortex:** The cortex lies between the medula and cuticle. It contains the melanin that gives your hair its color. The shape of the cortex determines whether you have straight or curly hair.
- **Cuticle:** This is the outer layer of your hair. It's made almost entirely of keratin. When magnified, the cuticle layer looks like a series of overlapping scales. These scales are the "armor" that protects the delicate interior of your hair from damage. It locks the moisture in and keeps bad stuff out.

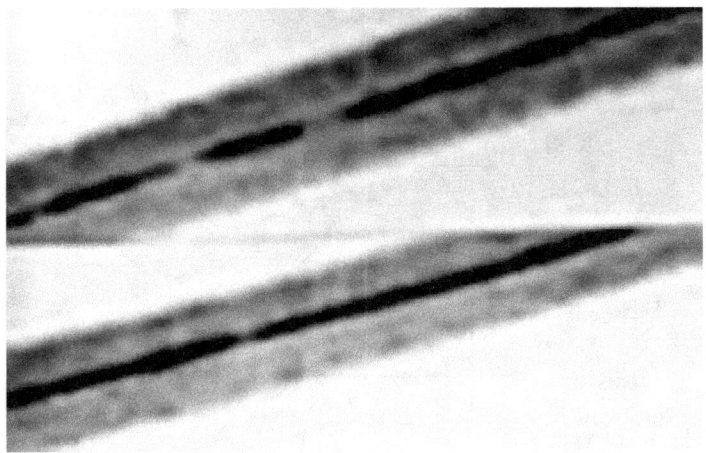

Figure 1: Hair with fragmented (top) and solid (bottom) medula.

Each strand of hair has three parts. The *root* is the part of the hair that's still beneath the skin. The *shaft* runs from the root to the *tip*, which is the portion of your hair that's the furthest from the root.

Let's take a quick look beneath the skin to see what happens as hair forms. Here's a picture showing a strand of hair beneath the surface of the skin:

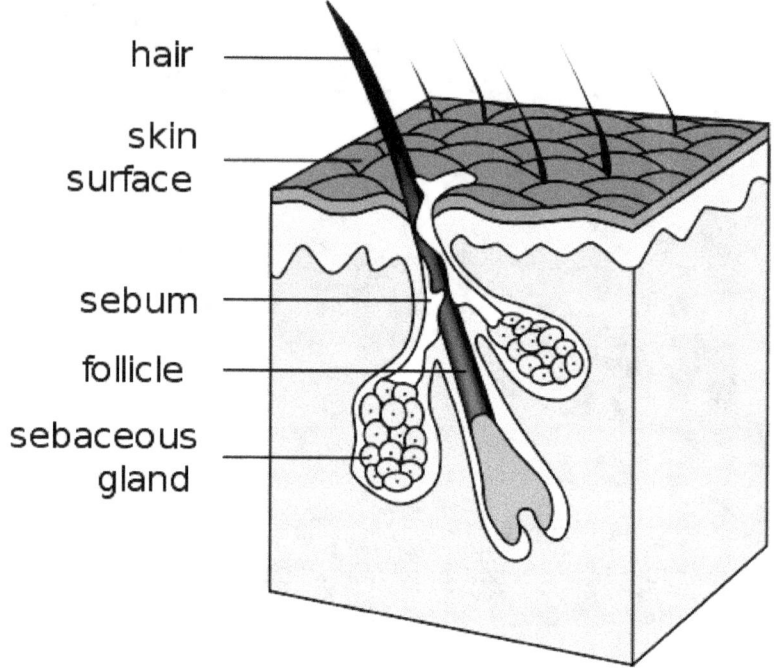

hair

skin surface

sebum

follicle

sebaceous gland

Figure 2: Hair above and beneath the skin.

A strand of hair begins forming in the *follicle*, which is located in the dermis layer of the skin. The *papilla* sits at the base of the follicle. This is the only living part of a strand of hair. The cells in the papilla divide rapidly and push the strand of hair up out of your skin. As the cells leave the papilla, they die and become keratin.

Hair grows in three distinct phases:

1. The *anagen phase* is the first phase of growth. It's the phase in which a strand of hair does most of its growing. It lasts anywhere from a couple years all the way up to eight years. Some people have longer anagen phases than others. That's why some people are able to grow their hair out to amazingly long

lengths while others have hair that seems to stop growing after it reaches a certain length.

2. The *catagen phase* is a brief phase that follows the anagen phase. It lasts for up to a month. The hair stops growing and the follicle begins to contract. The hair eventually detaches from the follicle and is pushed away from it as the follicle begins to deteriorate.

3. The *telogen phase* is the final phase of the hair growth cycle. It follows the catagen phase and lasts for up to four months. The follicle rests and rebuilds during this phase, preparing itself to start a new growth cycle. The strand of hair remains attached, but it doesn't grow. Once this phase ends, the follicle goes back into the anagen phase and starts growing a new strand of hair. The old hair falls out and the cycle starts all over again. That's why you end up with a bunch of hair on your brush and you may find some on your pillow from time to time. Losing up to 100 strands of hair a day is considered completely normal.

All of the hair on your head is in one of these three growth cycles at any given time. About 3% of the hair on your head is in the catagen stage and around 8% is in the telogen phase. The rest of your hair is in the anagen, or growing, phase. Your hair will grow approximately 6 to 7 inches a year.

There you have it. You're now an expert on the biology of human hair and its growth cycles. OK, you might not be an expert, but you know a lot more than the next person. That's got to count for something, right?

Bear with me a little longer; we're almost done with the scientific stuff. There's one more item we need to discuss— the sebaceous gland.

Sebaceous glands are found near the surface of the skin, usually attached to hair follicles. Their sole purpose in life is to emit *sebum*, which is an oily secretion that is designed to lubricate the hair and skin. The sebaceous glands add sebum to the hair and the hair transports it to the surface of the skin.

If you don't wash your hair for a few days, you might notice it starts to feel thick and greasy. If this happens, you have overactive sebaceous glands. In extreme cases, too much sebum can cause blockages in the follicle and will eventually cause you to have weak hair that grows slowly.

What You Need to Know About Curl Patterns and Hair Types

When it comes to natural hair, people tend to want to fit all naturals into a specific curl pattern or hair type. There are lettering and numbering systems out there that will tell you you're a 4C or a 3A or whatever the system thinks you may be. I've seen heated arguments break out between people arguing about what hair type they think they are.

The reality is you're probably not going to get much mileage out of trying to figure out your hair type or curl pattern. For one, there are literally tens of thousands of pictures out there of people claiming their hair is one pattern or another and there's no real way to tell who's right and who isn't.

You can post pictures on some sites on the Internet and the so-called "experts" will tell you what your hair type is. These posts often turn into big arguments where the self-proclaimed experts fight amongst each other as they try to determine your hair type. It's tough to tell from a picture what type of hair a person has.

You can go into a salon and ask the stylist to determine your hair type, but even then you're at the mercy of the individual stylist. I've seen cases where one stylist tells a person they have a certain curl pattern and another stylist tells her something different later on down the road.

The truth is it really doesn't matter what your hair type or curl pattern is. You have to figure out what works best for you. That's part of the journey. There are way too many variables to try to shoehorn a person into one particular hair type or pattern or another.

What I suggest is going to see a professional and asking what they think will work best for your hair. Forget about typing and patterns. Ask that he or she take a look at your hair and make specific care recommendations. They may not be 100% accurate, but they should give you a place to start.

Instead of spending countless hours researching hair types, spend your time testing new items in your hair and determining what works best in your particular case. Searching for your hair type can take a lot of the fun out of going natural. In the end, it's your journey. You determine the outcome—not some lady in a forum who may not know what she's talking about.

Porosity

The one thing you should be concerned with in regard to hair type is the *porosity* of your hair. Porosity is the amount of tiny holes there are in your cuticle layer.

Hair with high porosity has more holes in it and is going to be able to absorb moisture faster, but it's going to lose it faster as well. The cuticle scales on high porosity hair are lifted up and there are often gaps between the scales. This is the result of years of damaging treatments and harsh weather. Highly porous hair is hard to manage and often looks dull, dry and lifeless.

Hair with low porosity is the exact opposite of high porosity hair. It's going to be slow to absorb moisture, but will retain the moisture it does absorb for a longer period of time. If your hair has low porosity, the scales on the cuticle layer are tightly knit and they lay flat to the surface of the hair. This type of hair is considered healthy. It has luster and shine and flows nicely.

There's an easy test you can do to determine the porosity of your hair. Take a single strand of hair and drop in a pan filled with water. If it sinks within a minute or two, your hair is porous and will require extra care. If it's still floating after about 3 minutes, your hair has low porosity and is in good shape. Hair from different areas of your head may have different levels of porosity. Check hair from the front, back and middle of your head and check a couple hairs from along the edges. That should give you a pretty good idea of where you stand.

The porosity of your hair may change over time—and it usually won't change for the better. The only way to make damaged hair less porous is to grow out new hair and cut off the porous hair. Your new hair should be in better shape unless you have naturally-porous hair—then it isn't going to matter what you do.

How to Go Natural

Deciding you want to go natural is only half the battle. Once you make the decision to go natural, you've got to decide how you want to go natural. Transitioning to natural hair is the hardest part of going natural and it's the main reason people give up and go back to relaxed hair.

There are a number of ways you can choose to go natural. It's up to you to figure out which way best fits your lifestyle. You have to find the method that's right for you and is the one you're most likely going to be able to see through to completion.

Let's look at the various ways you can go natural.

Grow Your Hair Out

Growing it out is the least invasive method of going natural. You simply stop relaxing your hair and let it start growing out.

Going natural by growing your hair out lets you keep your hair at its current length while you grow out your natural hair. For women who can't imagine life with short hair, this is probably the best option.

Another benefit of this method is it allows you to slowly get used to your new natural hair. It will grow out slowly, giving you time to experiment with hair care products and styles to see what fits you best. You can take your time learning these things because your hair will grow out slowly. This allows you to stop using relaxer while continuing with your current hair care process until your hair starts to grow out. You get to ease into natural hair slowly but surely.

In addition to easing yourself into natural hair, you get to ease those around you into it as well. While the big chop can be jarring, growing your hair out allows you to slowly make the transition. This gives your loved ones and coworkers time to come to terms with the fact that you've decided to go natural.

This process is minimally invasive, but it's a long process.

You have to wait for your hair to grow, then trim a small portion of the relaxed hair off of the end, and then wait for it to grow again. Everyone's hair grows at a different rate, so there's no telling how long it will take. The average person's hair grows about a half inch per month.

Eventually, your hair will have grown out long enough for you to have trimmed all of the relaxed hair off. At this point you will officially be all-natural.

While this method may sound easy, there are some difficulties you need to be aware.

Your relaxed hair is going to have a different look and feel than the new, untreated hair that's growing out. This makes it tough to manage because the ends of your hair will be straight, while the new hair growing out is going to kink and curl. The relaxed portion of your hair will be weaker than the natural portion. The relaxed ends are going to be brittle and will break off easily if they aren't handled with care.

When you grow your hair out, the point at which the relaxed hair and the natural hair meet is called the *line of demarcation*. This line is difficult to manage because it can be pretty obvious. Twists, Bantu knots and braid-outs will be your best friend because they can be used to effective hide the demarcation line.

A natural hair softener can be applied to soften up your natural hair and make it more supple and manageable. This will help minimize the demarcation line.

You want to avoid hairstyles that require heat because heat will further damage and dry out your relaxed hair. If you have to wear your hair in a hairstyle that requires the use of heat, you need to limit it to once or twice a week.

You're going to have to handle your hair with care while you're growing it out. Wash and deep condition your hair at least once a week. Air drying is best whenever possible.

This will help prevent your hair from drying out when you hit it with the blow dryer. If you find yourself in a situation in which a blow dryer is necessary, you need to keep it at its lowest setting.

Natural hair is *porous*, which means it's able to readily absorb moisture, but it just as easily loses it. You have to constantly monitor your hair and add moisturizer to it when it needs it. Steer clear of chemical moisturizers. The natural ones are a much better choice. After adding moisturizer, add oil to it to lock the moisture in. This will keep the moisture in the hair shaft, where it belongs.

Try to avoid using a comb or pick to detangle your hair. A much better option is to rub some coconut oil into your hair and then detangle it with your fingers. Run your fingers through your hair and when you come to a knot you can gently pull it apart. If you use a comb or pick, you're going to damage your hair by trying to pull right through the knot.

Start at the end and untangle the knots closest to the end first. This allows you to easily pull them apart. Slowly work your way up until you reach the scalp. You're going to want to do a section of your hair at a time to make sure you get all of the knots.

Here is the five-step process for going natural by growing out your hair:

1. **Decide that you're going to grow your hair out and commit to making it happen.**
2. **Trim off the damaged ends of your relaxed hair.** You want to be sure to get rid of any split ends. Cut a half-inch or so off at a time for best results.

3. **Let your hair grow out.** As your hair grows, either trim it yourself or go have it trimmed at least once a month. Keep your hair in styles that minimize or eliminate the use of heat. The only time heating your hair is beneficial is when you're using heat while deep conditioning it.
4. **Wash your hair at least once a week and deep condition it.** You can use natural hair softeners during the conditioning phase if you'd like.
5. **Continue growing and trimming your hair until all of the relaxed hair is gone.** Pat yourself on the back. You made it!

Dreadlocks

If you have coarse-textured hair, *dreadlocks* might be a good option for going natural. With dreadlocks, you simply get your hair started binding and let nature take its course. As your hair grows out, the kinks and twists in your hair will interlock with one another to create your dreadlocks.

Dreadlocks are one of the easiest hairstyles to manage. Once you've got your hair locked up, you can throw away your combs and brushes. All you have to do is wash your locks periodically and you'll be good to go. You may want to trim them up occasionally, but that's entirely up to you.

You're probably going to have to get rid of your relaxed hair to properly start dreadlocks. The good news is you can start your locks with a little as an inch or two of natural growth. You can grow your natural hair out for a month or two, then cut off all the relaxed hair and get your dreadlocks started.

Starter locks are the dreadlocks you create in the beginning stages. If you plan on starting locks in hair that's shorter than a couple inches, you're going to want to use a tool designed to get dreadlocks started. The following methods can be used to start your locks:

Back combing. This is one of the more popular ways to dreadlock hair, but in my opinion isn't the most effective. It ends up doing a lot of damage to your hair and can hurt if someone else is doing it for you and they aren't careful. To backcomb your hair, you have to divide your hair up into sections and quickly comb it back towards the scalp so it mattes up. Wax or other products are used with this method to help the dreadlocks stay in or they tend to fall out when you wash them for the first time. Steer clear of wax and other unnatural compounds. You can add a bit of aloe vera gel if you want to help your hair lock up while backcombing.

Interlocking. If you want clean, neat looking dreadlocks, you can purchase a tool designed to make hair into dreadlocks. These tools can be used on all hair types and will form dreadlocks that are tightly locked with few loose hairs flying free.

Wool rubbing. You can rub a piece of wool around on your head until it causes your hair to matte up. This creates unpredictable patterns and can look messy.

Crocheting. This method involves using a felting or crochet needle to literally destroy your hair in order to get it to lock up. It can create nice looking dreads right away, but leaves your hair damaged and broken. This method is really bad for your hair and isn't recommended. There are actually support groups out there for people who have used this method and destroyed their hair.

Au-natural. Stop brushing and combing your hair and let it naturally lock up. This method is also known as the *neglect method*, because you leave your hair alone and let it do its thing. This method is the method to use if you want natural-looking dreadlocks that have the most energy. There are going to be loose strands and kinks and curls everywhere, especially during the beginning stages. There's a common misconception that this method takes longer than the other methods of forming dreads. It really doesn't, and there's something to be said about letting your hair go completely natural and watching it form its own dreads.

Twisting. Grab a section of hair and twist it between your fingers until you've got it twisted up enough so it stays together. Wait a week and touch your dreadlocks up by re-twisting the areas that are coming loose. Continue re-twisting at least once a week until the locks are able to hold on their own. This method can be used on extremely short hair. Be careful not to twist your hair too often or you can damage it and actually cause yourself to start losing hair.

Rip and twist. Pick out a section of hair. Twist it up between your fingers. Split it into two random pieces and quickly pull the two pieces apart. This will create knots that are pulled down to the base of the strand of hair. Continue this process of twisting, separating and pulling until the entire strand of hair is knotted up into a dreadlock. Rinse and repeat.

Braid and grow. Braid your hair in three-strand braids. Tie it or rubber band it at the end and let it grow out. The area that grows out will lock up. One the locked portion of your hair gets to be a few inches long, you can cut off the braids and grow the dreadlocks out. This allows you to keep your hair looking neat and is one of the only dreadlocking methods you can use that allows you to keep your relaxed hair.

Get it done. If you don't know what you're doing, it can be tough to get your hair to lock up properly. There are people who specialize in doing just this. Going to a professional will give you a good start. You also have the added bonus of being able to consult with the professional as to the best way to care for your hair and you have someone to call if problems arise.

Palm-rolling. This method entails rubbing a patch of hair together between your palms to get it to thatch up. This method doesn't work very well and doesn't last long enough to make it worthwhile.

Perms. I'm only including this method for the sake of completeness. I don't recommend it because it requires use of harsh chemicals to set your hair in dreadlocks. You're going "natural," so naturally you're not going to want to use chemicals to form your dreadlocks. That wouldn't make much sense. The chemicals used in dreadlock perms can cause permanent hair loss and balding and can actually prevent new hair from re-growing. You could be stuck with your damaged perm permanently.

You're going to want to avoid using wax on your dreadlocks. It's a popular way to lock up hair, but it isn't conducive to healthy hair. Wax pushes water and soap away, while attracting dirt and sometimes even bugs. It can also cause mold and mildew to grow in your hair, creating a smelly, stinky mess. If you've ever walked past a person with dreadlocks and been able to smell them from ten feet away, they probably use wax.

Dreadlock Maintenance

While there's no doubt dreadlocks are the most low-maintenance natural cut around (other than maybe going completely bald), you're still going to need to do some upkeep. You can't leave your locks alone to grow free and unchecked unless you want a dirty, itchy head full of mold and bugs. Unattended dreadlocks can get downright ripe in a short period of time.

Washing dreadlocks is easy. When dreadlocks are new, don't apply shampoo directly to the locks. Apply the shampoo to your head instead and let the water and soap run down them to wash them. Later on down the road once the dreadlocks are established, you can wash the locks themselves.

Steer clear of the shampoos that leave residues in your hair, regardless of what you may read on the Internet or on the label of a bottle that claims to be a "dreadlock" product. You want a shampoo that isn't going to leave a residue behind.

If you want to go all-natural with your hair cleaning products, you can use a baking soda/apple cider vinegar mixture to cleanse your dreadlocks. Create a baking soda rinse by mixing baking soda and water and apply it to your scalp. You can add a few drops of essential oil to the mix if you want your hair to smell good. Let it sit for 15 minutes, then wash the baking soda away. Next, add a couple tablespoons of apple cider vinegar to a cup of water and rinse your hair out with that. Once you're done, use clean water to wash the apple cider rinse from your hair. Using a baking soda rinse followed by an apple cider rinse should leave your dreadlocks soft and supple. If you want even healthier hair, try adding a few drops of tea tree oil to your baking soda rinse.

Depending on how greasy and oily your hair gets, you may have to wash your hair once a week—or you may be able to get away with doing it once every couple weeks or even once a month. You need to pay attention to your hair and scalp and wash it as needed.

Keep an eye on the base of each dreadlock. Locks tend to want to combine with one another. If you see this happening and don't want thicker locks, pull them apart regularly. If you do want thicker locks, be careful not to go too thick. Extremely thick locks can hold water and are prone to molds and mildews. Adding a bit of tea tree essential oil to your shampoo or cleanser can help prevent mold from forming.

Dreadlocks and Lice

There's a common misconception out there that dreadlocks are more prone to lice than other hair types. This isn't the case. You aren't more likely to get lice with locks. You aren't any less likely, either.

If you do get lice, you aren't going to be able to use the normal lice treating shampoo and the little comb that combs out all of the eggs. The good news is there are much better options out there for treating lice anyway. You don't have to put toxic poisons in your hair to kill lice. You just have to put something in your hair that suffocates them. 70% rubbing alcohol is your best bet, but you can also use petroleum jelly or mayonnaise. Neem seed oil is another good option that kills both lice and their eggs.

No matter what method you use, you're going to want to leave the substance in your hair for at least 20 minutes. Lice can survive without breathing for 15 minutes, so a 20 to 30 minute suffocation period should be more than enough. Place a shower cap over your head to keep the fumes in and further promote the die-off. It's going to take repeat treatment every 2 days for a couple weeks to completely eliminate lice.

You're also going to need to treat your bedding and furniture or you risk reinfection from your environment. Lice can live for up to 5 days without a host to feed off of.

The Big Chop

No single act elicits more fear and trepidation in the natural hair community than The Big Chop. The Big Chop is the process of cutting all of your relaxed hair off, so you can begin your natural hair journey with a fresh head of natural hair. When you Big Chop, you jump right in the deep end. Since there's no turning back, you need to be sure this is what you really want.

You're entering unknown territory and you're doing it without a safety net. For some, this is a liberating experience. For others, it can be a terrifying journey. You have to be willing to dive in headfirst without knowing exactly what's in store for you. Each journey is a different one and you can't predict what your hair's going to do. As long as you're prepared to not be fully in control every step of the way, you can handle the Big Chop.

In a way, you're telling the world "Here I am in my full natural glory. Love me just the way I am." Be prepared for a wide range of reactions. No hairstyle elicits more comments and a stronger reaction from people than the Big Chop.

If you're seeking instant gratification and are filled with a burning desire to go natural as soon as possible and with very little transition time, the Big Chop is the way to go. You jump from relaxed hair to natural hair in no time at all.

When you decide to do The Big Chop is up to you. You can cut it all off, let your hair grow out an inch or two before chopping it back or you can let it grow out 4 to 6 inches.

It's your journey; it's up to you to decide what the best option for you is.

In order to do The Big Chop yourself, follow these directions:

1. Part your hair into 4 even sections. You want to part it by dividing it in half from front to back, then splitting it again from ear to ear.
2. Divide each of those areas into 4 equal sections and place a rubber band or hair tie on each section just below the line of demarcation.
3. Cut off your relaxed hair below the line of demarcation. You want to get rid of all of the relaxed hair.
4. Once you've trimmed it, double check to make sure you got all of the relaxed hair. If not, trim the hair you missed off.

This method may create uneven lengths of natural hair because all of your hair isn't going to have grown at the same rate. If you want even hair, find the section of hair with the least amount of natural hair beneath the rubber band. Set all of your rubber bands at that length and cut the section of hair off at the band.

If you aren't comfortable doing this and are scared of messing it up, you might be better off getting it done by a professional. If you make a mistake, there's no turning back. You'll have to either cut it even shorter or wait for your hair to grow out.

The Teeny Weeny Afro (TWA)

The *teeny weeny afro (TWA)* is what you're typically left with after doing The Big Chop. You have an inch or two of natural hair left (if you're lucky) and you're left wondering what the heck you can do with it to keep it looking good and to keep you looking cute.

Some women opt for wigs until their hair has grown out enough to put it up in different hairstyles. I don't condemn anyone who goes this route, but to me it defeats the purpose of going natural. You want the world to accept you in your natural state—there's no need to cover it up with a wig.

Another option natural women often turn to is adding a touch of color to their hair. If you like dyes and don't mind using them, you can dye your hair brown, blond or any other color your heart desires. Just be aware dyes are harsh and can be tough on natural hair. You're going to have to really take care of your natural hair to keep it in good shape after dyeing it. Natural dyes like henna are a better option, but your colors are going to be limited.

There are a number of ways you can make your TWA look good.

Some women look great in their natural glory. Add a touch of curl enhancer and rock it in its full, natural beauty. I've seen a number of women who look absolutely radiant wearing this style. You can coil your hair up with some gel and a comb or you can twist it up if it's a little bit longer. Make it really shine by adding some coconut oil to it. Last but not least, you can add cute accessories like hair clips and bows to add a feminine touch.

How to Avoid Spending a Small Fortune

The natural hair care products sold in stores aren't cheap. When you're first embarking on your natural journey, you might find yourself wanting to try all of them. You're going to see multiple products recommended online and by friends and family members who have natural hair. You're going to be tempted to try all of them, not wanting to miss out on the best products out there.

What you're going to find out real quickly is that recommendations from others are almost completely worthless. Just because someone else endorses a product wholeheartedly doesn't mean you're going to love it as much as they do. I don't have any proof of this, but I suspect some of the hair care product companies pay people to go out and comment on blogs and seed posts into forums recommending their products. I've seen products recommended over and over again that I know don't work as advertised.

I'm an outspoken advocate of using natural products in natural hair. After all, the whole point of going natural is to stop adding chemicals to your hair to relax it. The next logical step is to stop using chemicals altogether. There are natural hair care products you can buy from the store that work great, but they cost a pretty penny. You're much better off making your own at home for pennies on the dollar.

Spend a lot of time with natural hair and you're going to see a lot of trends come and go.

As a rookie in the game, you're going to be tempted to jump on every new trend or treatment that shows its face. If you're onto something that's working for you, don't switch up your routing just because there's something new on the market that other people like. Be smart, and don't waste hundreds of dollars on new trends and unproven technology. Don't be a guinea pig. Give new items and products some time on the market and keep a close eye on what people are saying about them.

It also helps to remember that reviews can be faked. If a product has all glowing reviews and no detractors, it may be that the owner of the site deletes negative reviews in order to get more sales. Amazon.com is one of the better places to check reviews because they leave up both good and bad reviews and you'll get a (slightly) more objective view of the products you're interested in.

Another place you might find yourself spending a lot of money is at the salon. New naturals are excited about going natural and the ones who are growing their hair out instead of doing The Big Chop tend to go to the salon for trims more than they need to. Once a month is all you really need to go. Unless your hair grows really fast, you could probably get away with going every couple of months.

Keep an eye on the ends of your hair to judge when you need to go in and get a trim. Once you start seeing a lot of split, damaged ends, it's time to go get them trimmed. Don't run off to the salon the first split end you see. You're going to make them rich. If you really want to save money, you can keep an eye on your hair and cut any split ends you see off yourself. Save the salon for those special days where you want to try out a new hairstyle or you really want to look good.

When you do go to the salon, get a cut that's going to last. You don't want something that's only going to last a day or two unless you're going to a wedding or a funeral—or somewhere else where it's important to look your best. Even then, there are attractive hairstyles you can get that'll last you a lot longer than a day. Considering you might spend upwards of $50 on a styling session, you want to stretch your dollars over as many days' worth of hot hair as you can.

Take Care of Your Natural Hair

You need to have a hair care system in place so your hair doesn't get neglected. You best bet is to set up a weekly and monthly hair care schedule that you stick to the best you can.

It doesn't have to be difficult. Most people with natural hair only need to do the following things to keep their hair nice and healthy:

- Pre-cleaning (*pre-poo)* conditioning.
- Clean it.
- Condition and moisturize it.
- Deep condition and add protein.
- Seal it.

Everyone's hair is different and needs different amounts of each of these 5 items. Pre-poo conditioning should be done every time you clean your hair. You may find that you only need to clean and condition your hair once every couple of weeks while adding protein and deep conditioning it once a month. On the other hand, you hair may require a good cleaning and conditioning once a week and a deep conditioning with protein added every two weeks.

It's going to take some adjusting in the beginning. I'd start with weekly washing and moisturizing. Add protein and deep condition your hair once a month. Seal it every time you do anything to it.

You want to keep the products you use to a minimum. Use natural products whenever possible and try to use only a single product for each of the steps.

You may even be able to use one product that knocks out a couple of items at once. A moisturizing shampoo that cleans and conditions eliminate three steps with one product. You can save money, but the multi-tasking product may not work as well as three individual products that are tailored to each of the steps.

Once you've found a system that works, stick with it rigidly. Unless your hair changes and you need to make adjustments, there's no reason to mess around with a good thing.

Pre-poo Conditioning

Pre-poo conditioning prepares your hair for cleaning. It's up to you how far you want to take it. Some people don't bother with this step at all. Others claim it results in softer and suppler hair and they swear by it. I'd say it's probably a good idea to pre-condition your hair before washing and conditioning it. It isn't going to hurt.

The pre-poo stage consists of a couple tasks. You need to detangle your hair and then put something in it that prepares it for shampooing.

Detangling can either be done with a wide-tooth comb or your fingers. Rub some coconut oil into your hair to make it more manageable. The oil will reduce the chance of you doing damage to your hair while you get the knots out. Choose a small section at a time and work from the end of each section of hair to the base, removing all knots as you go.

Finger detangling is the safest way to go because you can stop when you get to each knot and pull it apart without doing too much damage. When you use a comb or pick, you rip right through the knots which can result in hair breakage and split ends.

There's no need to use expensive products for your pre-poo treatment. Whatever product you put in your hair is going to get washed out when you shampoo it anyway. Your pre-poo routine should be something that gets the cuticle ready for the shampooing and any treatment that is forthcoming. Treat your hair with your pre-poo conditioner an hour before shampooing it. Cover your head with a shower cap and leave the conditioner in until it's time to shampoo. Some people leave their pre-poo conditioner in their hair overnight and wash their hair in the morning.

The following oils can be used individually or you can combine them and use them as a pre-poo conditioner:

- Avocado oil.
- Castor oil.
- Coconut oil.
- Grapeseed oil.
- Jojoba oil.
- Extra virgin olive oil.

Heat up the oils that are solid until they melt and massage them into your hair and scalp.

In addition to oils, you may want to add other items to your pre-poo routine. Here are some items people have added to good effect:

- Aloe vera.
- Apple cider vinegar.
- Avocado butter.
- Cheap conditioner. If you have old conditioner you bought but didn't like, you can add it to your pre-poo conditioning treatment.
- Coconut milk.
- Egg whites.
- Glycerin.
- Honey.
- Plain yogurt.
- Shea butter.
- Cocoa butter.

No matter what you decide to add to your hair, it's important to test it on a small section of your scalp first. Wait at least 8 hours to make sure there isn't an allergic reaction. If there is a reaction, discontinue use of that item or product immediately.

Cleaning Your Hair

How often you clean your hair is something that's entirely up to you. You're going to see websites and books that tell you to wash your hair once a week, once every couple of weeks and even once a month. What I tell people is to pay attention to their hair and wash it when it needs to be washed.

If you have greasy, oily hair, you might find you have to wash it every few days. Once a week is probably the most common frequency at which people wash natural hair. Some people only wash their hair once every couple weeks or even once a month. I recommend washing it weekly because it gets rid of all the accumulated toxins and hair products and is more conducive to a healthy head of hair.

It's up to you to determine when you need to clean your hair. It's also up to you to determine which products work best to clean your hair. Every head of hair is different and is going to respond differently to different products. That's why you see online reviews of hair care products where some people love them and some people absolutely hate them. It's not that the products are good or bad; it's because they aren't as effective for some people as they are for others. A product that leaves one person's hair feeling thick and greasy may be exactly what another person is looking for.

Don't be afraid to try out new products, especially in the beginning stages of your natural hair journey. You're going to find products you like and products you don't like. As your hair starts to grow out, you may find that the products that worked great in your shorter natural hair don't work as well with longer hair. You need to be open to change in order to find out what works best for you.

Use a conditioning shampoo even if you plan on using conditioner in the next stage of cleaning. You can't condition your natural hair too much and using a conditioning shampoo isn't going to hurt your hair. It'll prime your hair for conditioning in the next stage.

Here are the steps you need to follow in order to clean your hair:

1. If you pre-treated your hair, remove the shower cap and use your fingers to detangle any big knots. If you detangled your hair during pre-poo treatment, this should be quick and easy.
2. Rinse the pre-poo conditioner out of your hair completely using lukewarm water. You want to rinse your hair for approximately 5 minutes to make sure you rinse everything out.
3. Use a gentle shampoo to wash your hair. Work the lather into your scalp. You have to make sure you clean your scalp really good because oils and toxins can build up on the scalp and cause all sorts of problems.
4. Work the shampoo into the rest of your hair.
5. Completely rinse the shampoo out.

That's it. Other than washing the pre-poo conditioner out, this stage isn't any different than what you've probably been doing to clean your hair for years.

Go Sulfate-Free

You want to avoid shampoos with sulfates in them.

Sulfates are *surfactants* designed to remove oil from your hair. At first glance, you'd think this was a good thing. The problem with sulfates is that they're harsh and can remove too much moisture from both your hair and your scalp, leaving you with irritated skin and dried-out hair. Not exactly what you want from a hair care product, is it?

If you're buying your shampoo over the counter (OTC), check the label and make sure none of the ingredients listed contain the word "sulfate." Common sulfates include sodium sulfates and ammonium sulfates. Sulfates are common in shampoos, so it may take a bit of searching before you find a good one that's sulfate-free.

Using sulfate-free shampoo is especially important if you plan on washing your hair more than once a week. The cumulative damage caused by sulfates can wreak havoc on your scalp and hair.

Why pH Matters

When you pick a shampoo, you need to take a look at the pH balance of the concoction and make sure you get one that's in the range of 4.5 to 6.5. The pH value of your shampoo tells you whether it's an acidic or a base liquid.

Both your hair and your skin can be negatively impacted if you use a product that has the wrong pH. You aren't going to find products that fall below 4.5, but you might see some that are above 6.5. Avoid these products, as they can cause frizzy, unmanageable hair.

Cleaning Your Natural Hair Naturally

I'm going to let you in on a little secret the hair care industry doesn't want you to find out about:

You don't need expensive shampoos full of the latest and greatest chemical compounds to clean your hair.

Sure, they work to clean your hair, but they also bathe your hair and scalp in an unnecessary bath of chemical compounds. These compounds can enter your body through your pores, and they stay in your body for a long time, doing who knows what.

You may be aware that most shampoos contain mineral oil. The name makes it sound like it's something good. After all, the body needs vitamins and minerals to survive. Well, mineral oil isn't what you might think it is. It's a byproduct created when crude oil is turned into gasoline. It coats your hair and gives it an artificial sheen. It also builds up over time, creating a thick oil slick that collects dirt and grime and prevents your scalp from releasing oil.

There are much better options for cleaning your hair. Natural options that aren't full of harsh chemicals and detergents. Two of the best natural items to clean your hair with are baking soda and apple cider vinegar.

We talked earlier about pH and why it's important you use a balanced shampoo. Baking soda and apple cider vinegar are completely natural and they balance one another out on the pH scale. Baking soda is slightly alkaline, while apple cider vinegar is acidic. You get the best of both worlds in an all-natural pH-balanced solution.

First, make a solution consisting of two tablespoons of baking soda mixed into two cups of water. If you have thick hair, you might want to add another tablespoon or two of baking soda. Don't be afraid to adjust the amount of baking soda to suit your needs. Add the baking soda and water to a container with a lid and shake it up until it's completely mixed. Wet your hair, and then massage the baking soda solution into it starting with your scalp and working your way out. Keep massaging it for a minute or two and rinse it out.

It may concern you that you don't get the suds you normally get with store-bought shampoo. The suds are added for effect and don't make your hair any cleaner. They're an unnecessary ingredient added to hair care products because they sell better when they foam up.

Baking soda is actually going to get your hair cleaner than most shampoo because it *clarifies* your hair, meaning it removes the gunk that builds up over time when you use chemical shampoos and hair care products.

Once you've washed the baking soda solution out, follow it up with a solution made of two tablespoons of apple cider vinegar mixed into two cups of water. Work a little bit of this solution into your hair, let it sit for a few minutes, and then gently wash it out. It will condition your cuticles and balance out the rise in pH caused by the baking soda.

When you first start using these two solutions, you might find that your appears to be oilier. That's because your hair has grown accustomed to having to produce extra oil to compensate for all the oil that's been stripped away by the harsh surfactants in regular shampoo. It might take a couple weeks for your hair to adjust, but it should eventually stop producing the excess oil.

If your hair continues to be too oily after a couple weeks, cut back on the amount of vinegar you're using and see if it helps. If your hair is too dry, try using honey instead of vinegar.

Conditioning and Moisturizing

There are two types of conditioning you need be aware of. Normal conditioning should take place every time you wash your hair. Deep conditioning is a heavier form of conditioning that should take place around once a month. This section covers normal routine conditioning. We'll get to deep conditioning later.

Conditioning is an important step in the natural hair care process and shouldn't be skipped. You should condition your hair every time you clean it. This becomes especially important if you're using store-bought shampoos that strip hair of its natural moisture.

Natural hair is prone to drying out and needs to have moisture added back to it regularly. Natural oils aren't able to travel down a length of naturally-curly hair the way they can down straight hair. Your natural hair needs your help to stay moist, and that help comes in the form of conditioning.

Conditioning should be done after you shampoo or otherwise wash your hair. Follow these instructions to properly condition your hair:

1. Divide your hair into 4 to 8 sections depending on how thick your hair is.
2. Rub conditioner through each of the sections of hair. Be sure to completely coat your hair with conditioner.
3. Detangle your hair while the conditioner is still in it.
4. Rinse the conditioner out.

Leave-in Conditioner

You can optionally apply a *leave-in conditioner* designed to be left in your hair. This will add even more moisture to your hair.

Leave-in conditioners are light sprays or lotions that are applied to your hair after you wash and condition it. You rinse out your hair, apply the leave-in conditioner and then leave it in your hair.

These conditioners aren't designed to replace normal conditioners. They are to be used above and beyond any conditioners you may normally use. They add moisture and help seal it into the hair by covering any holes there are in the cuticle layer of your hair.

Natural Conditioner

There are a number of recipes out there for natural conditioner and I've tried most of them. Some have worked and some have left my hair feeling sticky and greasy. I don't condemn any of them. Like I've said before, natural hair is a personal journey and you need to find the right product for you. What works great for me may not work at all for the next girl.

My personal favorite is to mix one whole egg with half a cup of plain yogurt and then massage it into my scalp. I always rinse conditioner out with cold water in order to further seal the cuticles. It leaves my hair feeling nice and soft for days after I've used it.

In addition to eggs and plain yogurt, the following items can be used to help condition your hair. Mix and match them as you see fit and play around with the amounts you use to see what works best with your hair:

- Olive oil.
- Jojoba oil.
- Lavender essential oil (only use a few drops, as this is powerful stuff).
- Rosemary essential oil (only use a few drops).
- Coconut oil.
- Tea tree oil (only a few drops are needed).
- Seaweed.
- Argan oil (just a little).
- Honey.

Be sure to wash any natural conditioner you use from your hair as completely as you can before moving on to the next step.

Deep Conditioning and Adding Protein

You should deep condition and add protein to your hair at least once a month. I've seen some literature that recommends doing it once a week, but I think that would be a bit much for most hair types. Once every two weeks to a month will be more than enough to add in the extra moisture your hair needs. *Deep conditioning* is similar to regular conditioning in that it adds moisture back into your hair, but it does so much more aggressively.

It's expensive to go to the salon to have it done. I've heard of places charging as much as $50 a session to treat natural hair. That can get pretty expensive if you're going once every two weeks. The good news is you can deep condition your hair at home and save a lot of cash.

When you deep condition your hair, you can skip the conditioning step. Wash your hair with a moisturizing shampoo, rinse it and then go straight into deep conditioning. You want to completely coat your hair with deep conditioner. Once you've coated your head, you want to cover it and let it sit for 30 minutes.

For best results, deep conditioning needs to be combined with heat. You can use a heating cap or a hooded dryer if you have one. If not, you can set your hair dryer on low and use it maintain a constant stream of warm air on your head. Just make sure you don't get it close enough to melt whatever it is you have covering your head. Even if you don't get burnt, you don't want to spend hours trying to remove melted plastic from your hair. Keep moving the hair dryer around and hold it as far away from your head as you can. To be honest with you, it's not really worth the risk when you can get a heating cap for 30 bucks that'll get the job done.

Here's a trick you can use until you get your heating cap. Wash your hair and apply deep conditioner to it. Throw a shower cap over it and stay in the shower for a little while, letting the heat of the shower warm up your head. This isn't ideal, but it'll work in a pinch.

Hair steamers are another item that work well with natural hair. You add deep conditioner to your hair and put on the steam cap, which then proceed to keep your head warm and moist using steam instead of just heat. Hair steamers are more expensive. A good steamer will run you around a hundred dollars.

Regardless of what method you use, heat your hair for 30 minutes to get the conditioner to really set in. After the 30 minutes is up, detangle your hair and rinse the conditioner out.

Natural Deep Conditioning Treatments

The best part about doing deep conditioning yourself at home is you can use all-natural ingredients that work as good, if not better, than the products used by salons. You can also do it for pennies on the dollar. An at-home deep conditioning will only cost you a couple bucks.

Here's an all-purpose recipe you can use to make your own natural deep conditioner:

- 1 ripe banana, mashed
- 1 ripe avocado, mashed
- 1/4 cup coconut milk

- ¼ cup Shea butter, melted
- 3 tablespoons honey
- 1 egg
- A few drops of your favorite essential oils for scent and added benefits

If your hair needs extra hydration, add a couple tablespoons of extra virgin olive oil or a quarter cup of aloe vera gel. Mix all of the ingredients in a food processor or blender until completely incorporated. Apply it the same way you would store-bought deep conditioner.

Protein Treatment

Protein treatment adds protein to you hair. If your hair is in good shape, you can get away with a light protein treatment that you can do at home. On the other hand, if your hair is brittle and breaks easily, you may need a more aggressive treatment done at a salon.

Light protein treatments can be purchased over the counter. They can be applied as often as once every couple weeks, but if your hair is healthy there's no good reason to do it more than once a month. Protein treatments on their own can cause your hair to become brittle, so you should always balance them out with a moisturizing conditioner.

At-home protein treatments will have little to no effect on badly damaged hair, especially if the damage comes from overuse of chemicals products. These treatments should be done at the salon under the supervision of a professional. Don't get them done more than once every couple of months and only then if you're experiencing severe breakage problems.

CHI sells a keratin mist you can spray on your hair daily to provide your hair the protein it needs. This is a preventative mist that can be used to help alleviate problems later on down the road. Apply it after showering and leave it in your hair for best results.

Seal It

The last step in the hair care process is *sealing* your hair. When you seal your hair, you apply an oil or butter to it that locks moisture in the hair shaft. Without a sealing oil, your hair is going to dry out a lot faster. 100% yellow Shea butter or almond oil are good choices for sealing your hair.

The reason your hair dries out when it isn't sealed is because of the scales in the cuticle layer. There are gaps between each of the scales on the surface of your hair. When you moisturize your hair, the moisture enters through these gaps (so does dye when you dye your hair). The problem is the moisture leaks right back out in a short period of time. The more damaged your hair is, the more holes there are in the cuticle layer for moisture to escape from.

When you use a sealing oil or butter, the oil or butter fills in the gaps in the cuticle layer, slowing down the escape of moisture. Eventually the oil or butter will wear away and the moisture will escape, but it takes a lot longer for your hair to dry out than it does when no sealer is applied.

Always seal your hair as the last step in your hair care process. Sealing your hair earlier in the process locks moisture out instead of locking it in.

How to Grow Long Natural Hair

Early in your journey you may decide you want to keep your natural hair short. It's easier to work with and easier to clean when it's short. You're also limited as to what you can do as far as hairstyles go and a lot of women don't care for short hair. If you're anything like the average woman with natural hair, you want your short hair to grow out as soon as possible.

A lot of naturals turn to vitamin B7, or *biotin*, to try to speed up the growth of their hair. Some women swear by it, claiming it their hair began growing rapidly once they started taking it. All scientific evidence points to this being false, and the women who think it makes their hair grow may have experienced a placebo effect. Regardless of whether it works or not, you should be getting more than enough in your diet.

I've heard stories of women taking mega-doses of biotin to try and stimulate hair growth. This may pose health risks and you need to discuss the appropriate amount of biotin you should be taking with a medical professional prior to starting to take it.

Taking good care of your hair will help it grow longer. If you create and stick to a hair care plan that encompasses all of the items discussed in the last chapter, you'll be able to grow your hair out longer because it will be healthy and less likely to break off before it reaches its full length.

I'm now going to tell you something you probably aren't going to want to hear. Genetics play a huge role in how long you're going to be able to grow your hair. If you've had thin hair that's impossible to grow out since birth, there isn't much you can do to change it. You can take steps to make your hair stronger and healthier, but there isn't much you can do to add more hair to your head or to make the hair you do have grow longer. Growth cycles determine the length of your hair. If you have short growth cycles, your hair isn't going to grow out nice and long.

Now for some good news. Genetics play a huge role in hair growth, but your genes aren't the only player in the game. There are other elements at play as well, some of which you may not be aware of.

Diet and Hair Growth

Diet is another contributing factor, and it's a big one. While genetics ultimately determines how long your hair grows and how full of a head of hair you're going to have, your diet may be holding your hair back from reaching its full potential.

You need to eat a healthy, balanced diet to ensure your hair gets the nutrients it needs to grow. The following ten items should be included in your diet to help your hair reach its maximum potential:

- **Green veggies.** Green vegetables like broccoli and dark, leafy greens are packed with vitamins conducive to healthy hair growth.
- **Legumes.** Beans are packed with protein. You already know how good protein is when applied to your hair. It's also good for your hair when you eat it.
- **Carrots.** Carrots are full of vitamin A, which is good for your skin and scalp.
- **Dairy.** Milk, yogurt, cottage cheese and other low-fat dairy products add protein to your diet. Dairy also contains calcium, which is another item your hair needs to remain healthy.
- **Eggs.** Eggs also add protein to your diet.
- **Lean meats.** More protein.
- **Nuts.** The zinc in nuts has been shown to keep your hair on your head where it belongs. Not having enough zinc in your diet can lead to excessive amounts of hair falling out. Walnuts are especially

beneficial because they contain Omega-3 fatty acids that other nuts don't have.

- **Fish.** Salmon, herring and tuna all have high levels of Omega-3 fatty acids that are used to create your hair.
- **Oysters.** These shellfish contain high levels of zinc and protein.
- **Blueberries.** This superfood helps the body in a number of ways, one of which is providing the body with nutrients needed to grow a healthy head of hair. If you aren't including blueberries in your diet, you should be.

Adding these foods to your diet and eating a balanced diet can help your hair reach its full potential. If you aren't eating right, you could be stunting your hair's growth.

Drink More Water

Adding moisture to your hair from the outside is important. It's also important to add it from the inside. You do this by drinking more water. You can use the best of the best products in your hair and eat all the right foods and still derail your efforts at gaining a healthy head of hair by failing to drink enough water.

How many cups of water do you drink daily? One? Two? None? It might surprise you to find out that most people need at least 8 cups of water a day to stay healthy. Some sources say men need as much as 13 cups a day and women need 9 to 10 cups a day.

And no, soda, juices and other beverages don't count.

So, what can you do if you can't stand the taste, or lack thereof, of water? You can spruce it up with a slice of citrus fruit or you can drink herbal tea. Those both count toward your daily water intake.

Drinking more water promotes healthy skin, which in turn helps your hair grow because the follicle gets all of the moisture it needs. Drink water to maximize your hair's growth potential.

Turn Down the Heat

Blow drying, hot curling and using a flat-iron are all good ways to damage your hair by drying it out. When you apply heat to your hair, you cause what little moisture your hair does have inside to evaporate.

This can leave your hair feeling dry and brittle. The more heat you use, the worse off your hair will be. Dry, lifeless hair that breaks easily is often the result of overuse of heat while styling. Too much heat can even damage the natural curl of your hair, leaving it looking lifeless and resting flat against your head in some spots while puffing out in others.

Keep your heat styling to a minimum and set your devices to the lowest setting. For example, instead of curling your hair every day, wear it in styles that don't require heat during the week and only curl it when you go out on the weekend. You won't completely eliminate heat by doing this, but you'll cut the days you use it from 7 days a week to one or two days a week. Or you can find cute hairstyles that don't require heat and completely eliminate it. Your call.

One source of heat a lot of people fail to take into consideration is the heat of the water being used for showers or to bathe in. Some people like their water right on the verge of scalding the skin off their bones. If you're one of those people, your hair may be suffering because of it. Water that's too hot can damage both your hair and your scalp, hitting you with a double whammy that may be thinning out your hair.

Your hair will be shinier and healthier as a result of turning down the heat. You'll also have less split ends. The only time heat is good for your hair is when you use it during the deep conditioning stage.

Ditch the Dye

Thinking about dyeing, bleaching or highlighting your hair? Better think twice.

Bleaching damages your hair on multiple levels. It dries your hair out and makes it more porous than it was before. What this means is even if you add moisture back to your hair afterword, it isn't going to stay there. Leave the bleach in for too long and you're at risk of making your hair so porous that it can no longer hold together. Prolonged exposure to bleach can make your hair brittle and give you what's called a *chemical haircut*. Bleach agents can also burn your scalp if they come in contact with it.

Permanent dyes bathe your hair in a bath of damaging chemical compounds. They're designed to break through the cuticle layer of your hair in order to create color that's vivid and lasts a long time. Every time you dye your hair with permanent hair color, you create more and more perforations in the cuticle layer. While these tiny holes are great for letting the dye in, they aren't so great when it comes to keeping moisture in the shaft of your hair where you want it.

If you dye your hair yourself at home, make sure you follow the instructions on the box to a T. Don't leave the dye on your hair longer than instructed "just to make sure." It's not going to work any better; it's just going to cause further damage to your hair. Even if you follow the instructions exactly as they're written, you're going to do damage. Leaving the dye in your hair causes even more damage than normal.

It's going to cost more, but you're probably better off going to a stylist and getting it professionally done. A good stylist can keep damage to a minimum and will give you the best dye job with the least amount of damage done.

Temporary dyes don't do the same damage, but they have to be applied frequently. These dyes coat the cuticle layer without punching through it. While they're easier on your hair, they aren't really a good choice because they have to be reapplied after every washing.

All-natural henna dye is a good option for those looking to avoid the pitfalls of chemicals dyes while using a dye that's going to last more than a couple days. Henna dye lasts from 30 to 90 days before it has to be reapplied. Test it on a small patch of hair the first time you use it because it can cause an allergic reaction.

Clarify Regularly

Clarifying your hair means taking steps to make sure you remove the build-up of old products, dirt and grime from your hair. When you use OTC products, each time you use them a little bit of residue is left behind. This residue builds up over time, leaving behind an oily, greasy mess that leaves your hair feeling heavy and matted.

You can use a clarifying shampoo designed to rid your hair of residue. This method works, but the clarifying shampoos are rather harsh and contain chemicals that can damage the structure of your hair if you use them too often. You should only a clarifying shampoo once a month if you decide to go this route.

There's really no reason to use clarifying shampoo. The baking soda/apple cider vinegar treatment in the chapter on cleaning your natural hair naturally is one of the best clarifying treatments around. Just to review, you wash your hair with a baking soda solution, and then follow it up with an apple cider vinegar solution for good measure. These two solutions combined will clarify your hair and get rid of any build-up effectively and naturally.

Swap Your Hair Care Products Out

It also helps to switch up your hair care products every once in a while. Your hair becomes conditioned to a product when it's used repeatedly over a long period of time and the effectiveness diminishes.

To combat this, try to find two to three products you like for conditioning and to use as shampoo and rotate between these items. Make the swap every other month for best results. That way, you keep your hair guessing as to what's going to be put in it and it won't become immune to any one product.

Take Your Hair Out of Traction

Wearing your hair in hairstyles that constantly pull on the scalp and the hair follicle can cause permanent damage. Tight cornrows, braids or even putting hair ties or rubber bands in too tight can cause all sorts of issues, up to and including hair loss and premature baldness.

The scientific term for hair loss associated with too much traction is *traction alopecia*. It's common amongst women with natural hair because we tend to wear our hair in styles where too much pressure is placed on the follicle. The more the hair is pulled on, the greater the potential for contracting traction alopecia becomes.

We've all seen the old (and many not-so-old) ladies in our community who are losing their hair or who have large patches of skin exposed on their scalp. This baldness can often be attributed to traction alopecia.

While you usually can't reverse traction alopecia once it's happened, you can take steps to make sure it doesn't get worse. Loosen up your braids, cornrows and twists a bit to relieve pressure on your scalp. Wear your hair in looser styles to avoid pulling it out by the root.

Don't Over-Moisturize

You're going to see book after book and website after website talk about how important it is to moisturize your hair. I've even seen literature that claims you can't over-moisturize your hair. I'm about to shoot holes in that theory. You absolutely can have too much moisture in your hair.

While it's important that you don't let your hair dry out to the point that it's brittle and breaks easily, you also don't want it to be so damp and moist that it looks like you've got a Jheri Curl all the time. There has to be a happy balance.

Hair with too much moisture looks damp and feels limp to the touch. It may also feel stretchy like a rubber band. A little bit of elasticity in your hair is good. Too much elasticity is a bad thing because it allows your hair to stretch to unnatural lengths. When you stretch healthy hair out, it rebounds back when you let go of it. Over-moisturized hair stretches, but fails to rebound back.

If your hair feels like it has too much moisture, cut back on the frequency of your deep conditioning and conditioning sessions. If you're conditioning once a week, try cutting back to once every couple of weeks. Deep conditioning can be cut back as well. Another way to combat over-moisturizing is to up the frequency of your protein treatments. Protein treatments with hydrolyzed proteins and amino acids will give you the best results.

Protective Styling

Protective styling is defined (at least by me) as any hairstyle that protects your hair from harsh conditions and harm. Hot and cold weather, snow and rain, wind and sun. Your hair takes a beating. Add in hairstyles that pull on your hair unnaturally and daily styling that includes brushing and heating and you've got a recipe for disaster.

A protective styling gives your hair a break from your rigorous daily regimen while largely protecting it from outside harm. The intent is to allow your follicles and your hair a break from the daily routine. Your protective hairstyle protects your hair from further damage during this break.

Protective styles are more often than not styles you put in your hair and leave in for as long as you want your hair to be protected. You can sometimes go for months with a protective hairstyle with minimal maintenance required. It gives both you and your hair a much-needed break.

Braids and twists are considered protective styles as long as they aren't too tight. You want them to be nice and tight, just not so tight that they are on the verge of pulling your hair out by the roots. They can be left in for long periods of time and require little to no maintenance. Braid and twists that are to be used as a long-term protective style need to be kept on the smaller side because the bigger versions tend to frizz out and need more maintenance. One trick you can use to keep your hairstyle looking fresh is to redo the braids or twists along the edges of your hairline once every couple of weeks. This will keep you looking nice and will prevent the loose hair from starting to lock up.

If you only want to protect your hair for a day or two, you can put it up in a bun or simply cover it with a hat or a scarf. These are quick and easy protective styles that you can put on in a jiffy.

Anything that tucks the fragile ends of your hair out of sight is technically considered a protective style. The ends of your hair have been around the longest and have sustained the most damage. Keeping them tucked away in a protective style protects them from further damage. Try adding a bit of leave-in moisturizer to your ends before you hide them away.

How often you wear a protective hairstyle is up to you. If your hair is dry and damaged, you may want to wear one for a few months to allow new, undamaged hair to grow out. Those with otherwise healthy hair might opt for protective styling only on days where the weather is going to be particularly nasty—or you might choose to wear a protective style here and there to preemptively give your hair a break from the norm.

Keep washing to the bare minimum necessary to keep your hair clean. Twists will usually last a couple washings, while braids can last as many as 4 or 5 washings. The less you wash, the longer your hair will be protected. You also want to avoid unnecessary use of hair styling products. A true protective hairstyle won't require you to use any product at all. Here's a tip that should help your hairstyle last through an extra washing or two. Braid your braids or twists into larger braids before washing them. This will add an additional layer of protection to your hair.

Detangling

We briefly touched upon detangling in an earlier chapter, but this is a topic that warrants a closer look. You're going to have tangles and you're going to need to get them out. There are a handful of methods being used by naturals to get the knots out of their hair. We're going to take an objective look at the methods that actually seem to work and it's up to you to try them and see which one is best for your type of hair.

Natural hair tends to be fragile and is easy to damage, so ripping through dry hair with a comb or brush isn't a good option. You may be able to use a wide-tooth comb to detangle wet hair, but you're going to want to be careful. Going too fast can make minor knots worse and cause your hair to break when you try to force your way through it. Some people are lucky enough to be able to use a comb without causing problems. Others aren't so lucky.

For women with sensitive or damaged hair, finger detangling is a better option, albeit one that takes significantly more time that using a comb. When you use your fingers, you're more likely to detect knots in your hair before you pull them into one another and make them worse. Using your fingers lets you feel out each knot individually and then pull it gently apart.

Regardless of whether you're using your fingers or a comb, you're going to want to separate out a small section of hair at a time. Start at the end of a section of hair and detangle it from tip up. Getting the knots closest to the end out first prevents you from pulling knots that are further up in the section of hair into knots that are below it. Separate one knot at a time as you work your way up and your hair will be all the better for it.

Some women prefer detangling their hair when it's dry. Fine, thin hair is usually easier to detangle dry. Others prefer detangling when their hair is wet or damp. The most common way to detangle natural hair is to add a bit of conditioner to it first. You can also add oils or butters to it to help your fingers slip through the strands.

Be careful not to stretch wet or oiled hair too far. It's going to be elastic and highly flexible. Make sure you don't stretch it out too much during detangling or you might have breakage issues once it dries out a bit.

The 7 Biggest Reasons for Excessive Hair Breakage

There are a lot of reasons your hair might be breaking off before it reaches its full potential. Hair breakage is the number one reason women with natural hair suffer from thin hair and short lengths that we can't seem to improve upon. Eliminating the following 7 items from your life— and from your hair—will go a long way toward solving your problems with breakage.

7) Permed Hair

The chemicals used in perms are a known carcinogen. That alone should be reason enough to avoid perms. They're also extremely harsh chemicals designed to break down your hair at the molecular level. Natural hair is inherently weak. When you get a perm, you're further weakening the structure of your hair and opening it up to more breakage. Avoid perms at all costs. If you have hair that's already damaged from excessive perming, your only option may be to grow it out.

6) Dye

Permanent hair dye strips your hair of its natural color and replaces it with the new color. It leaves your hair dry and brittle in the process. Every time you dye your hair you stack more damage on top of the damage caused by previous dye jobs until your hair can't handle it anymore and starts breaking off.

5) Traction

Pulling your hair too tight puts undue stress on your hair. Traction alopecia occurs when your hair begins breaking off at the root. Too much traction weakens your hair and can permanently thin your hair out.

4) Sleeping on cotton pillowcases

While the previous three items are common knowledge amongst women with natural hair, this one isn't as well known. The pillowcases you're sleeping on may be damaging your hair while you sleep. Cotton pillowcases wick moisture away from your hair, leaving it dry and brittle. The same thing goes for cotton hair accessories like scarves. Invest a little bit extra and go for silk pillowcases or tie your hair up in a silk scarf before you go to bed. A silk pillowcase won't absorb moisture and oils and it allows your hair to effortlessly slide across its material.

3) Your hair care products.

The stuff you put in your hair could be drying your hair out and causing problems with breakage. Hair products that are petroleum-based and contain mineral oil block moisture from getting into your hair. They also build up on your scalp and aren't conducive to hair growth. You get the double whammy of breakage combined with slow growth when you use petroleum-based products.

Products with ethyl alcohol dry out your hair. This type of alcohol is found in styling products designed to hold your hair in place. Double check the labels on your hair care products to make sure you aren't unknowingly drying out your hair.

2) Lack of moisture

Dry hair is brittle hair. If you have dry hair, you need to condition your hair regularly to add moisture. Once you've added moisture, you need to seal it in by applying oil. Badly damaged hair is porous and water leaks from it in a number of places. Applying oil temporarily plugs at least some of these holes. Condition and seal your hair every time you wash it to ensure it has the moisture it needs.

1) Too much combing or brushing

It's important that you detangle your hair (unless you're trying to get dreadlocks to form). Combing or brushing your hair excessively puts pressure on the roots and damages the shafts of your hair, especially if you aren't careful. Keep combing to a minimum and steer clear of brushes altogether.

Most people either have done or currently are doing a number of the items on this list. If you're doing just one of these items, you're causing damage to your hair that could result in breakage. Those of you doing more than one are going to be doing even more damage. You're at risk of doing permanent damage and by the time the effects start to show, it may be too late.

I wish I would have had this list when I started my journey. At one point of time, I was doing all 7 of the items on the list at the same time. I'm lucky my head of hair survived without any visible permanent damage. Other people aren't so lucky. We've all seen the ladies that don't appear to have even edges along the edge of their hair. That can usually be attributed to breakage.

Thin Edges

Thin edges aren't something that happens overnight. Sure, genetics plays a role in how thick and alive your edges are, but most people start with a decent amount hair on their edges. Over time, the cumulative effect of many of the items discussed in the previous chapter can contribute to thinning edges.

The number one cause of thin edges is too much stress being put on the hair. We've mentioned traction alopecia a few times now. The edges of your hair is where it usually starts because when you pull your hair too tight the most pressure it places on the hair along the edges.

For a lot of us, excessive pressure on our edges started from an early age. Our mom would braid our hair up real tight before school or pull our ponytails so tight it felt like our eyebrows were lifted up. Tight hair sits flatter to your head, so it's easier to pull your hair tight when you're putting it in a ponytail, a braid or any number of other hairstyles.

Extensions are another contributing factor to thin edges. Good stylists are very thorough and will make sure they include every last hair when putting extensions in. Ask them to go easy on your edges and you'll be much better off in the long run.

To prevent thin edges, keep your hair moisturized and avoid pulling it too tight. Styles like braids, buns and puffs need to be kept to a minimum. If you put your hair up in styles that put stress on the edges frequently, you're going to want to wear protective styles from time to time to give your edges a break.

Avoid hair care products that contain alcohol and keep the chemicals you add to your hair to a minimum. If you need to use styling gel, your best bet is to use one with aloe vera gel in it instead of alcohol.

Natural Remedies for Thin Edges

The first thing you need to do when you notice your edges starting to thin is to stop whatever it is you're doing that may be contributing to it. None of the natural remedies in this chapter will have a chance to heal your hairline if you continue to damage it. To be completely honest with you, they may not work at all if the damage is bad enough, but it's worth a shot.

If you notice your edges are starting to look a little rough, you might be able to bring them back by putting your hair into a protective style that keeps pressure off the edges for a few months. Avoid anything that pulls your hair tight and you might see your edges start to fill back in.

Jamaican black castor oil is castor oil before it's gone through the refinement process. It's powerful stuff that's capable of removing toxins from your scalp. Massage it in once a week to help your scalp properly make and release sebum.

Aloe vera is packed full of helpful vitamins and minerals. While it's found in a lot of products, there is usually only a small amount tossed in for good measure. Try rubbing aloe vera gel into your scalp to help unclog your pores and to provide a nutrient boost to your follicles. Aloe vera may not be able to reverse the effects of traction alopecia, but there is evidence that indicates it may help stop further hair loss.

There are a number of oils you can add to your hair care system that are thought to promote growth and healthy hair. Peppermint essential oil, grape seed oil and cinnamon essential oil are three of the more common oils. If you decide to use them, remember these are powerful oils that should never be applied to the skin at full strength. They have to be mixed with carrier oils like avocado or jojoba oil before application. It only takes a few drops mixed with carrier oil to treat your entire head.

As with any new product, test anything you try to help repair your thin edges on a small section first and wait 8 to 10 hours to see if there's an allergic reaction. You don't want to find out you're allergic to something after you've slathered it all over your head. Trust me on this one.

How to Fix Frizzy Hair

Frizz. It's the natural enemy of natural hair.

Everything will be going along just fine and one morning you wake up and your hair is frizzed out in every imaginable direction. Frizz is one of the main reasons women give up on their natural hair journeys. It's too bad, really, because frizzy hair can be controlled using a handful of common sense natural techniques.

There are a number of reasons your hair may be frizzing out and it's important you identify the right reason. You aren't going to be able to find a solution if you aren't sure what the problem is. While you can usually make an educated guess, it may take some trial and error testing to figure out what's actually going on.

One cause of frizzy hair is the pH balance of your hair. If the pH balance shifts toward the alkaline side, it can cause your hair to swell up and become unruly. If you're using alkaline products and your hair is frizzy you either need to discontinue use of the alkaline products or add something to your hair care regimen to shift your hair's pH back to the middle. If you're using the baking soda/apple cider vinegar rinse from the hair cleaning section and you still have frizzy hair, pH probably isn't the issue. It's time to move on to something else.

Here's a trick the seasoned vets use. Try coating your hair with a dark beer like Guinness and letting it sit for 10 minutes before rinsing it out. Dark beer will add moisture and nutrients to your hair and can help knock down frizz.

One of the biggest causes of frizzy natural hair is humidity. When the humidity goes up, so does the volume of your hair. This is a tough one to deal with because Mother Nature is tough to beat. Your best bet is to make sure your hair has all the moisture it needs before heading out for the day. Leave-in conditioner works wonders on days where the humidity is making your hair crazy. Treat your hair with conditioner, and then apply oil to seal the moisture in. This will also lock additional moisture out.

Here's another natural home remedy for frizzy hair. Apply mayonnaise to your hair, cover it with a heat cap and leave it in your hair for 30 minutes. Wash out the mayo and apply warm coconut oil to your hair and put the heat cap back on for another 30 minutes. Wash and clean your hair with cold water when you're done. The cold water will help seal the cuticles back up.

Here's another tip. Give your hair enough time to dry before you leave the house on cold, dry days and on humid days. If you leave the house with damp or wet hair, you're going to have frizzy hair by the time your hair dries. Let it dry, apply some Shea butter to it and you'll be able to make it through the day with a lot less frizz than you'd have if you washed your hair at the last minute and ran out the door with damp hair.

When all else fails, put your hair in a style that minimizes the effects of frizzing and wait it out. A cute scarf, headband or bow can be used to minimize frizzing, as can protective styles that pull your hair up like buns. If you have to have your hair in a style where frizzing is obvious, carry a small spray bottle full of conditioner or your favorite oil. When your hair starts to get unruly, knock it down with a few sprays from the bottle. It isn't an ideal solution, but sometimes it's the only thing that works.

Here's one last tip to help cut down on frizzing. Towel drying your hair can make it wild and unruly, especially if you're rough with the towel. Drip-dry your hair if you have time. If not, you should have a hood dryer on hand to speed up the process. Hood dryers are easier on your hair than blow dryers and won't make a mess out of your hair. They distribute the heat evenly across your head and free up your hands to do other stuff while your hair dries. They aren't as expensive as you might think. A good one can be purchased for around $60.

Natural Hair Styles

Let's wrap this book up with a look at some of the more popular natural hair styles. Contrary to what some people would have you believe, there are a lot of natural styles to choose from—and there are styles suitable for any and all situations and occasions.

We already discussed dreadlocks in the chapter on how to go natural, so I'm not going to rehash that information here. Click on the following link to go back to that section:

Go to Dreadlocks Section.

The types of hairstyles you have available to you depend on how long your hair is. If you have short hair, you're going to be fairly limited. If you have long hair, you're going to have a lot more options. Regardless of whether you have short or long hair, I'm sure there's a hairstyle that's right for you.

You might have to experiment and play around with a hairstyle or two—or ten—before you find one you're happy with. I've said it before and I'll say it again. This is your journey. If you aren't happy with something, don't be afraid to change it.

The Natural Fro

Let's start with the easiest natural hairstyle of them all: the natural afro. This and dreadlocks are the most natural styles there are. You're going back to your roots when you wear this style.

There's no single right way to wear a natural afro.

You can wear what's called a *wash-and-*go, which is exactly what it sounds like. You wash your hair and go out, letting it do what it wants to do. You can let it fly free, you can puff it out for more volume or you can add leave-in conditioner or oil to it to give it a fresh out the shower look. Try adding bows or a headband or you can pull it back in a puffy ponytail.

I don't recommend doing this all the time, but you can blow-dry your afro to add even more volume to it. Use a heat shield and use the blow dryer to blow your hair up away from your head.

The natural afro is a favorite hairstyle of many women because it's easy to rock and there are so many things that can be done with it. It's like the Swiss Army knife of natural hairstyles.

Afro Puffs

An afro can be pulled up into one or a number of *afro puffs*. Afro puffs are quick, easy and sassy. You can create as many puffs as you want. One big puff looks good, as do many smaller puffs.

To create a single afro puff, all you have to do is gather up the hair you want in the puff and put a hair band tight at the base of the puff. Fluff the hair in the puff out to make it appear puffier. To create multiple puffs, you do the same thing, but in multiple sections of hair. Divide the hair out first into even amounts and then create your puffs.

Twists and Mini-Twists

Twists are one of the more popular hairstyles for natural hair. That's because they're easy to do, they last a decent amount of time and they look good in almost any type of natural hair.

Figure 3: Simple two-strand twist.

Two-strand twists are the easiest twists to do. Follow these directions to create two-strand twists:

1) Pull your hair up and clip it so the hair on the back of your head is easy to access.
2) Start at the base of your neck and work your way up your head until all of your hair is twisted. You're probably going to want to enlist the help of someone else to do the twists on the back of your head until you're comfortable doing them.
3) Separate out a section of hair. How big of a section you separate out is up to you. If you want big twists, separate out a large section of hair. If you want smaller twists, separate out a smaller section of hair.
4) Divide the section of hair into two pieces of equal size.
5) Start at the scalp and crisscross each strand over the other one all the way up the length of hair. You want to pull the hair tight enough that it locks the two strands together.
6) When you get to the end of the section of hair, twist the ends together between your fingertips. If done right, the twist will stay in your hair without you having to put a clip or rubber band on the end.
7) Repeat the process until your entire head is complete.

Mini-twists are done the same way; you just use much smaller sections of hair. With mini-twists, your twists will look nice and tight.

The only product most naturals need to add to their hair is a 50-50 blend of Shea butter and coconut oil. Apply the mixture to each of the sections of hair before you begin twisting them.

While twists are easy, it's time-consuming to do your entire head. It can take 3 to 4 hours to finish twisting up a whole head of medium-length hair. Shorter hair can be finished in a couple hours.

The good news is your twists will last you a long time if you did them right. Twists can last as long as a couple months if you take good care of them. A good way to ensure the longevity of your twists is to sleep on satin or silk pillowcases or pull your hair up in a satin scarf before you go to bed.

Twists are a protective hairstyle that keeps your hair out of harm's way and gives you time to grow out healthier hair. When they're done right, they look professional enough that they can be worn anywhere.

You can play around with your twists to give them your own unique touch. One twist (pun intended) on this technique that I've seen done to good effect is to twist your hair up into about 15 twists in the evening before you go to bed. Use Shea butter when you twist them up and leave it in overnight. In the morning, remove the twists. You can leave them as-is or fluff your hair out for a poofier look. You can also add curlers to the end for even curlier hair.

Another play on the twist technique is to do your twists on dry hair. Add a little bit of butter and twist them up for a slightly different look. Twists done on dry hair will be longer than twists done on wet hair. You can really show off your length with dry hair twists.

If you have longer twists, you can pull them up into a bun or you can put them in a ponytail. You can also twist or braid your twists with each other. Twists also look great when pinned up.

Comb Coils

Comb coils are loose coils that give your hair a cute, curly look. You can do this style on all lengths of hair, from freshly chopped hair to long hair that's below your shoulders. It's easier to do on shorter hair, but don't let that stop you if you want to try it on longer hair.

Follow these directions to create comb coils:

1) Wash your hair, condition it and detangle it. Detangling is important because bad tangles can form during comb coiling if you haven't properly detangled your hair.
2) Part a section of hair out or pick a section out at random.
3) Add a dab of gel to the section of hair and spread it across the whole section.
4) Start twisting the section in one direction, starting at the base and working your way to the end.
5) Once you've got it twisted up tight, let go and it should spring out into a cute little coil.

Comb coils are quick and easy, but they don't last very long. You're lucky if you get a couple days out of your comb coils before they have to be redone.

Braids and Cornrows

Braids are a protective hairstyle you can put your hair in when you want to give it a break. They can often be left in for more than a month with minimal maintenance required. While you can braid shorter hair, it's easier if you have mid-length hair or longer.

There are a number of different braid styles you can do, but they're all based on the same basic premise. Here's what you need to do to braid your hair:

1) Wash and condition your hair.
2) Section it off and clip or band each section. The bigger the sections, the bigger your braids will be. If you want to keep it neat, use a rat-tail comb to make neat parts.
3) Pick out a section of hair and apply coconut oil, Shea butter or leave-in conditioner to it.
4) Detangle the section of hair, starting at the bottom and working your way up to the scalp.
5) Divide the hair into 3 equal portions. You'll have an outer-left piece of hair, a middle piece of hair and an outer-right piece of hair.
6) Take the section of hair that's on the right and put it under the middle section and over the left section. You'll once again have a left, right and middle section of hair. Repeat the process. Put the section on the right under the middle section and over the outer section.
7) Repeat this process until you reach the end of the hair.

8) Secure the end of the hair with a clip or a rubber band to keep the braid in place.

Cornrows are done in a similar manner, except you work from the front of the head to the back, keeping the braids tight to the head. Here are the instructions for doing cornrows. It's a little tough to explain how to do them in print, so you might want to do a search on YouTube and watch a few videos before you try this technique yourself. Once you get the hang of it, it's fairly easy.

Here are the steps required to cornrow hair:

1) Part out a triangular section of hair, starting from the front of the head and running to the back. You want the parts to be clean because they're going to be visible once the cornrows are complete.
2) Separate out a small section of your triangular section from the front of the head. You want the cornrow to start at the edge of the hairline. Add a butter- or oil-based holding cream to the section of hair you plan on working with. This will help keep everything in place as you go.
3) Divide the small section of hair into three equal pieces and make a few braids, keeping them tight to the scalp.
4) Add more hair to each of the three sections and continue braiding, keeping your braids tight to the scalp.
5) Slowly work your way toward the back of the head, adding more hair to each of the three sections as needed.

6) When you reach the back of the head, continue braiding the loose hair in the section until you reach the end of the strands of hair.
7) Put a clip or a band on the end of the cornrow to keep it in place.

It's easier to learn how to do braids and cornrows on someone else's hair first. Once you get good at it, you'll be able to do it on your own head, but you might need some help with the back.

Micro braids are another popular hairstyle. When you do micro braids, you create tiny braids that only use 20 to 30 strands of hair in each section of the braid. This creates thin braids that aren't much bigger than a single strand of hair. You can use micro braids in a number of other hairstyles. Try braiding micro braids into bigger braids for a unique look. One warning about micro braids—they take forever. You're going to need at least 4 or 5 hours to micro braid your hair, maybe longer.

The Ponytail

Some days you just don't feel like spending hours doing your hair. The ponytail is perfect for those days. It isn't going to get many oohs or aahs, but you can rock a ponytail when you're running down the street to grab something from the store and don't want to leave unruly hair flying free.

You can combine the ponytail with other styles. Braids and twists can both be pulled back into a ponytail. If you have shorter hair, you can put the hair in the back in a ponytail and twist or curl the hair closer to the front that won't reach the ponytail.

Gel bands without a seam are your best bet for a ponytail in natural hair. They don't get tangled up in your hair and are easy to put in and remove. The old-fashioned bands with the metal pieces on them need to be avoided at all costs. They damage your hair and can get badly tangled, especially if you fall asleep with one in.

Rod Sets

Flexi-rod sets leave your hair looking vibrant and curly. All you need are some flex rods, a bit of setting lotion and some Shea butter.

Here are the directions for doing a flexi-rod set at home:

1) Gather up a bunch of flexi-rods of various sizes.
2) Add equal parts setting lotion and water to a spray bottle.
3) Start off with damp hair.
4) Gather a 1-inch thick section of hair and rub Shea butter down the length of it.
5) Spray setting lotion on the section of hair.
6) Make sure there aren't any tangles.
7) Roll your hair up into the flexi-rod. Start from the end of your hair and roll it up to where your hair meets your scalp.
8) Fold the ends of the flexi-rod over so it holds the hair in place.
9) Let your hair air-dry. This can take up to 6 hours if you have long hair.
10) Remove the flexi-rods from your hair.
11) Separate the curls by pulling small sections of hair out of each curl. Twist the curl in the direction of the curl while pulling it away from your head. This step takes practice to get right. Play around with it to see what you like best. Add a small amount of olive oil to your fingers when you pull out your curls for best results.
12) You can fluff your hair out from the roots using a wide-tooth comb if the curls are sitting too flat.

Bantu Knots

Bantu knots are a great starter hairstyle that can be done on any length of hair. They're a protective hairstyles that can be used to put your hair up and keep it safe. You can even do them with dreadlocks without damaging the locks.

Here are the steps for creating Bantu knots:

1) This style can be done on wet or dry hair. You can add a bit of oil or leave-in conditioner to it to make it more workable.
2) Part the hair into even squares. You want the parts to be nice and clean because they'll be visible. A rat-tail comb can be used to create the parts.
3) Clip the sections of hair you aren't working with up out of the way.
4) Twist the hair at the base of where the hair meets the scalp. Continue twisting in one direction until it starts to wrap around itself. Continue to wrap your hair in this direction until you've formed a knot. The size of the knot depends on how long your hair is and how much hair you separated out for the knot.
5) Tuck the end of the hair into the bottom of the knot. Pull it snug so it won't work its way out.

Bantu knots will last for up to a week if you cover your head with a silk scarf when you go to bed. Once they start to unravel, you can either redo the knots or pull them all out and rock a wavy afro for a couple days. Either way you're going to look good.

Enjoy Your Journey

This is the end of this book, but only the beginning of your journey. Going natural is a life choice that's very rewarding. It can also be frustrating, especially during those times where your hair seems to have a mind of its own. Stick with it, and you'll come out the other end a stronger and better person.

I hope you enjoyed the book and learned a thing or two from it. I also hope you enjoy your journey. Keep your eyes peeled for more books in the Natural Hair Journey series. This is the first of a planned series of books on natural hair.

See you around…and when I do, I hope to see you in your all-natural glory.